Using your brain to get rid of your pain

A simple, common sense guide on how to manage stress, reduce pain, and think more healthily.

By John Perrier, Physiotherapist

Title and Copyright notice

"Using Your Brain to Get Rid of Your Pain"

A simple, common sense guide on how to manage stress, reduce pain, and think more healthily.

By John Perrier

Published by JP Publishing Australia

Copyright 2015 John Perrier

ISBN 978 0 9577-4041-9

Self Help/Relaxation/Healthy Living

Also available as an E-Book

ISBN 978-0-9875694-0-0

Please see the end of the book for:

More titles from this author

Ways to connect with us

Acknowledgments

My thanks go to Ian McKenzie, Psychologist (B.A.Hons, Psych, MAPS) of the Gregory Terrace Rehabilitation Clinic in Brisbane, for his comments and suggestions. Ian freely gave of the knowledge he has accumulated over ten years of working with chronic pain patients.

I would also like to thank Hilary Thompson, Occupational Therapist, for her comments and suggestions. Her work as the head of the relaxation clinic at The King Khalid National Guard Hospital in Saudi Arabia has provided her with a keen, practical sense of which techniques really work. Her suggestions were much appreciated.

I also acknowledge the work of Bert Weir, from the Relaxation Centre in Brisbane, whose work has already helped thousands of people.

Notes

#1. This booklet comes with a complimentary downloadable MP3 relaxation track. This audio track closely follows the methods outlined in this book, and will be a valuable aid to your learning and implementation of these techniques. To download it, please visit our web site and follow the links under "Using Your Brain to Get Rid of Your Pain".

#2. Much of the information in this book has been extracted from another work by the same author entitled *Back Pain - How to get rid of it forever*. It is available as a paperback, or as a two-volume E-Book. Please see our web site for more details.

www.JPpublishingAUSTRALIA.com

Table of Contents

Chapter One

"An introduction to pain"

An introduction to pain

Pain! No matter what type of pain you are suffering, I'll bet that you need no introduction. In fact, you probably know pain *too* well.

Your pain may be aching, searing, stabbing or burning. It might be a dull headache, crippling arthritic pain, an acute back spasm, a frustrating bout of the 'flu, or any one of a million other painful maladies. The episodes might be short and sharp, or continue unremittingly for weeks, months, even decades on end.

Whatever type of pain you are suffering, the techniques in this book will show you how to decrease its 'hurt'.

This book does *not* contain masses of hard scientific data or in-depth psychiatry. Nor is it a collection of old wives' remedies, religious doctrine or hippy-inspired new age alternatives. You won't be using drugs, needles, or special equipment, nor will you be required to burn incense, chant mantras or wear mystical healing crystals in a bracelet around your ankle. Instead, you will learn how to relieve your pain using the most natural cures known to medical science.

Furthermore, the treatment will have beneficial spin-offs rather than unpleasant or dangerous side effects. Better still, it won't cost you a single penny!

Please don't think that any of the information in this booklet implies that your pain is 'all in your head'. This is almost certainly false, and you should be wary of anybody who tells you so. In fact, the opposite is more likely to be true: you will soon see how stress causes real, measurable and identifiable changes in your body, which can cause a wide range of pain-provoking conditions.

Many maladies, such as headaches, stomach ulcers and heart attacks are so closely linked to elevated stress levels that relaxation techniques form an indispensable part of their rehabilitation. However, the benefits of stress reduction are not just limited to these types of conditions. You will find that principles in this booklet will even help to diminish pain that is totally unrelated to stress, such as a broken leg, or even a cancerous tumour.

In short, almost anyone with pain will benefit from learning and applying the principles outlined in the rest of this booklet. Some people will experience a complete cure. However, before you continue, please heed the following two pieces of common sense advice.

First, pain is a vital and necessary signal from your body, telling you that something is wrong. The pain-relieving techniques in this book are very effective – so effective, in fact, that they can mask potentially serious conditions. You should always consult an appropriate health professional who can properly diagnose and treat the underlying causes of your pain. *This information does not replace conventional treatment techniques - it complements them.*

Second, you should be realistic when assessing the role that your mind can play in both creating and curing diseases. Robert Sapolsky, a highly-regarded researcher and author on stress-related illness, summarises this notion perfectly when he says "Everything bad in human health is not caused by stress, nor is it in our power to cure ourselves of all our worst medical nightmares merely by reducing stress and thinking healthy thoughts full of courage and spirit and love." So please, don't expect overnight miracles. Nevertheless, I am sure that you will receive immense pain relief and other health benefits if you understand and practice the principles of relaxation and pain reduction.

Before we end this chapter, let me share with you some statistics that I find not only surprising, but a bit silly. A study in the United Kingdom investigated the attitude of public towards deep mental relaxation and hypnosis. The researchers put three questions to a large number of people with chronic pain, and tabulated their responses.

First, the subjects were asked a simple question: if their doctor recommended a tablet that would cure their pain, would they take it? One hundred percent of respondents said 'yes', they would take the tablet.

The researchers then asked the subjects a second question: if your doctor recommended that surgery would cure your pain, would you have the operation? Here, 65% of people said yes, 15% were not sure, while 20% said that they would refuse the surgery. Fair enough.

Finally, they were asked a third question: if your doctor recommended that hypnosis would cure your pain, would you undergo the treatment? Only 40% of people said that they would agree to be hypnotised, while 20% were unsure. Surprisingly, 40% of people would flatly refuse such a treatment, even though they trusted their doctor and knew that it would cure their pain.

Think about it. Compare the dangerous and painful consequences of surgery with that of deep relaxation and hypnosis. Yet many more people would accept the dangers of anaesthetic, tolerate post-operative pain, and endure hospital food, rather than have a few sessions of deep relaxation!

From where does this irrational fear arise? Is it a deep-seated mistrust of allowing another person to manipulate our minds? Is it a fear that we will be exposed as unable to cope by ourselves? I don't know.

Dr Ainslie Meares, a prominent Australian psychiatrist, has written of the reticence of many of his patients to perform simple relaxation exercises. He cites cases in which he spent many treatment sessions not teaching or practicing the exercises, but simply trying to convince the patient that they would work. Not only that, but even after the patient had reaped considerable benefits from the exercises performed in his surgery, many patients refused to continue them at home in front of their family or friends.

Again, I do not know why this attitude exists. However, this self-awareness is a very real problem for some people. My only advice is this: the sooner you start the relaxation exercises, the sooner this irrational feeling will go away.

I know that many joggers feel the same sense of self-awareness when they first start their exercise regime. Some runners feel very embarrassed during their first few attempts, believing that people are staring or sniggering at them. Nothing could be further from the truth. Be honest and straightforward about your exercises, and the benefits that you receive from doing them. You will soon discover how to relax your way to better health and a pain free life.

The human brain is a very complex system. Often, we aren't even sure how to use or control it, as the millions of people who suffer with anxiety, depression, or phobias will testify. Unfortunately, our brains didn't come with an instruction book, or an *on-off* switch.

Luckily, researchers from a wide section of the general and medical community have devoted themselves to uncovering better ways to control our thought processes. Over the next four chapters, you will learn these principles. You will....

(1) Discover how stress affects your body.

(2) See why some people are often sick, while other people are always healthy.

(3) Learn exercises that will decrease your stress and pain levels.

(4) Relieve your pain by altering how you think about it.

In learning these key areas, you will not only discover how to control your own stress levels and get rid of your pain, but you will experience the enormous benefits that come from a healthy and relaxed mind and body.

Now take a slow, deep breath, and then relax as you exhale. Repeat this deep, relaxing breath twice more before you continue reading. Are you feeling more relaxed already?

Chapter Two

"The effects of stress"

Why stress is worse than the bubonic plague, AIDS and the common hangover all rolled into one.

The effects of stress.

If the symptoms of stress were all the same, humankind would realise that we were dealing with a disease worse than the bubonic plague, AIDS, and the common hangover all rolled into one.

While doctors and other experts cannot precisely determine a figure, many feel that about 50% of all pains and illnesses in today's society are due, in some part, to stress. Others argue that this estimate is way too low. Why do we tolerate such a devastating plague with such seemingly little response from health practitioners?

One reason that stress-related problem receive such scant attention is that they do not present themselves as a straightforward diagnosis. Stress appears in many different forms, and underlies many seemingly unrelated conditions.

For example, if an elderly widow goes to the doctor with an upset stomach, she may be diagnosed with an ulcer, not with 'stress'. When a fifty-year-old executive presents with chest pain, he is diagnosed as suffering from angina, not from 'repressed anger'. And a housewife may be told she has dermatitis when she develops itchy skin, not 'anxiety'. Yet these cases, and thousands of others just like them, were probably caused or exacerbated by stress.

Similarly, when you see a health practitioner about your sore back or neck, they will usually examine your spine, not your mind. Fair enough, too. Yet while a joint or disc may be causing your current pain, it is possible that your high stress level over prior years caused your joints to degenerate in the first place.

Another reason that health practitioners often ignore stress is that it is so complex. When we talk about the causes of stress in the next chapter, you'll see that they are almost impossible to define as simple, identifiable situations. Because the reasons are hard to pinpoint, they are difficult to treat objectively.

These complications mean that medical and other mainstream health training facilities largely ignore training and research into stress management. Consequently, stress-related pains and illnesses are often handled poorly by all but a few dedicated practitioners. Often, the time is spent - for better or for worse - on more immediate problems and solutions. Stress is usually put into the too-hard file, which may help to explain why anxiety, tension and their related symptoms are epidemic.

In the next few chapters, you will learn about many aspects of stress, including how it causes pain, why it affects you, and how to decrease it. We'll also discuss some more abstract qualities of stress, such as how the power of the mind can help your total well being. I hope that the following discussion will, in some small way, help to counterbalance the lack of attention stress and relaxation usually receive from health practitioners.

But *I'm* not stressed

I wonder if at this point you are thinking 'I'm not stressed ... none of this really applies to me.' However, before declaring yourself as an island of calm, you should be aware that most people who are stressed don't even realise it. This unintentional ignorance occurs because stress builds so gradually and insidiously that you are usually unaware that it is happening.

Furthermore, the demands and pace of modern life mean that *most* people are stressed, and so we come to accept a high level of stress as normal. After all, if our parents and siblings are stressed, our work colleagues are stressed and our friends are stressed, then we don't even realise that we are uptight. Yet then we are surprised or annoyed when we fall ill, we suffer from repeated headaches, or our backs become sore for no apparent reason.

Another reason that you may not realise how much tension you are carrying is that chronic stress does not show itself in an obvious way. If you don't eat, you become hungry. If you don't drink, you feel thirsty, and tiredness will soon let you know if you've been missing sleep. However, your body is not so good at telling you that you should be relaxing. The signs can be subtle, varied, and sometimes nonexistent until it's too late.

For all of the above reasons, may people are simply unaware that stress is contributing to their problem.

Stress causes not only pain, but can also alter moods and attitudes, and can create physical changes in the body. As you read the following lists, count how many of these signs and symptoms are familiar to you.

Common effects of stress on the mind
- Alcoholism
- Apprehension
- Cigarette smoking
- Depression
- Drug dependence
- Fatigue
- Feelings of anxiety
- Headaches
- Insomnia
- Irrational fears/phobias
- Irritability, impatience
- Lack of motivation or energy
- Lack of concentration
- Short temperedness
- Obsessive behaviour
- Panic attacks
- Stuttering

Common effects of stress on the body

- angina, heart attacks, or irregular heart rhythms
- Arthritis
- Asthma
- Back pain, neck pain
- Cold sores, mouth ulcers
- Constipation or diarrhoea
- Fibrositis, aching joints
- Frequent bouts of the 'flu or other viral illnesses
- Migraines, stress headaches
- Sexual problems
- Shortness of breath
- Skin problems, itchiness, rashes
- Stomach dyspepsia, nausea, reflux or ulcers
- Tendonitis
- Tight muscles, trigger points (knots)

Anything sound familiar? If so, then my bet is that at least some of your pain is stress-related. So let's now look at the stress process in more detail, and discover how it affects your mind and body.

How does stress cause pain and illness?

You may be wondering exactly how stress causes physical aches and pains, as the relationship at first seems tenuous. Many people rightfully ask questions such as 'How does the tension/anger/anxiety that I feel toward my boss/partner/situation translate to pain arising from my heart/head/joints? The two problems seem so removed from each other.'

That's a very good question. Which has a very long answer.

Before we look at this answer, please be aware of one subtle but very important point: stress does not *directly* cause most of these conditions. Rather, *it decreases the ability of the body to resist* other agents that create these maladies. Also, stress *increases your chances of catching diseases or developing problems* that make you sick or cause you pain.

Unfortunately, this simple point – that stress exacerbates the intensity and frequency of illnesses and pain, rather than directly causing them - is frequently misunderstood. Perhaps this misunderstanding is why one health practitioner might insist that your problem is entirely due to stress, while another will dismiss this notion with a flippant wave of the hand, instead blaming a more tangible factor such as a virus, a blocked artery or a worn out joint.

Think of a stressful lifestyle as like driving without a seatbelt. Driving without a seatbelt does not *directly* cause you any harm, but it certainly increases your chances of being hurt if you have an accident. Furthermore, if you are unfortunate enough to crash while not wearing your seatbelt, you may, as I'm sure your parents forewarned you, 'crack your head open on the windscreen', and suffer a very serious injury. Of course, if you were properly restrained, the damage would not be as likely, and would probably also be less severe.

Likewise, if you are excessively stressed, you will not automatically contract a huge array of diseases and conditions, but rather you will be more likely to develop them. Additionally, the repercussions of any condition will probably be more severe than if you had a relaxed state of mind.

Nevertheless, the science of *pathopsychophysiology* – that's stressology to you and I – has postulated some well-proven ideas as to how anxiety and emotional tension affect the body. To appreciate these theories, and to comprehend the stress process altogether, you must understand a reaction called the *fight-or-flight* response.

The fight-or-flight response is a prehistoric reaction of the body to prepare it for battle - a fight - or to run away from danger - the flight. (Some researchers use another 'F' word to denote preparation for sexual activity, but as this is a family book, I'll leave that one out.)

When one of your prehistoric ancestors was faced with danger, its brain reacted in two ways. First, it activated a subconscious part of the nervous system, known as the *sympathetic nervous system*, to alter the function of various organs. These organs then changed almost instantly to prepare themselves for fight-or-flight.

Secondly, your ancestor's brain released hormones into its bloodstream. These hormones stimulated other glands, such as the adrenal glands, to release other hormones that further altered the body's function in preparation for sudden physical exertion. You are probably familiar with the effects of one of these hormones, adrenalin. Another substance released by the adrenal gland is called *hydrocortisone*, which you will learn more about soon. In short, the fight-or-flight syndrome causes the body's systems to prepare themselves for sudden physical exertion, diverting all of its energy into avoiding the present crisis.

These same stress responses persist to this day.

For example, the fight-or-flight syndrome channels your body's blood flow to your muscles to supply them with oxygen and energy that is needed for powerful movements. It causes your heart rate to accelerate and your respiration to deepen, preparing your cardiovascular system for action. Your pupils dilate to allow in extra light, and sometimes your hairs even stand on end in an outdated attempt to make you appear bigger and more fearsome. All of these responses are rapid, reproducible, and are automatically stimulated by the perception of danger.

During prehistoric times, these responses were appropriate. The fight-or-flight response played a vital role in preparing the body to avert danger. Without these reactions, our ancestors would have probably perished in the dangerous, hostile place that was prehistoric Earth.

However, the threat of physical danger is rare in modern society. Sure, most of us are concerned for our physical well being a few times during our life. However, most of us generally meander through life without the threat of being eaten by a dinosaur, or being scalped alive by a warrior from the tribe next door. But in today's society, these physical dangers have been replaced by another source of stress.

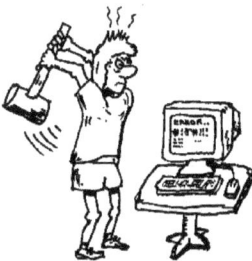

Computers.

Computers that break down. Computers with incompatible software. Computers whose hard drives crash on a regular basis, taking with them at least three chapters of this booklet that I have forgotten to back up. Did I mention computer keyboards that lose the 'E' key? (Ar you sur that I didn't mntion that bfor?)

Oh, and while I'm talking about stress situations, could I add 'when patients turn up late for appointments', and so plunging my carefully planned afternoon into disarray? Humid weather - I hate that, too. And people who drive slowly in the right lane. Worst of all is when the city council phone machine puts you on hold for twenty minutes, and then tells you to call back later. And paperwork. And meaningless registration fees. And....

Sorry about that rant, I got carried away. Can you see that although we no longer have many physical threats in our lives, that these dangers have been replaced by hundreds of new stress agents?

However, our body still uses the same old way of coping with stress: the fight-or-flight response. So guess what happens when (pick one that applies to you):

(a) Your parents come home from their holiday a day early. Unfortunately you had a few (hundred) friends around last night, and now have thirteen seconds to complete about nine hours of cleaning.

(b) You discover that your wife has thrown out your favourite 'Adam and the Ants' T-Shirt that you've kept since high school.

(c) Your overweight, leering boss, who has been looking you up and down since you started work in the typing pool, asks you to stay after work to help him with some 'urgent business'.

(d) Your baby daughter, who is now fifteen, is going out on her first date. Her partner, a scrawny, pimply seventeen-year-old with a bad moustache, picks her up in a panel van.

(e) You're late for an important meeting, and find yourself stuck on a single lane road behind a little old lady in a Lada. Even worse, she's wearing a bowls hat.

(f) Your toddler son has been screaming for two hours because you won't let him eat a bag of dry flour, and your three-year-old daughter refuses to release your leg until the neighbour's cat goes home. Your infant nephew is intent on pushing a lollipop into your ear. You still have to tidy the dining room, set the table, and make the soup before your guests arrive ... in eight minutes time.

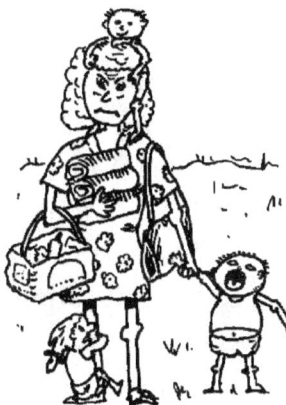

Can you guess what happens in these, or any one of a million other, stressful situations? That's right, *your body initiates a fight-or-flight response.*

Your sympathetic nervous system kicks into action, and adrenalin, hydrocortisone and a handful of other hormones are released into your blood. These physical responses to stress are so unambiguous and reproducible that they can be measured with a blood test. They cause your muscles to tense, your heart and breathing rates to increase, and make your pupils dilate.

In short, your body undergoes responses that would have been appropriate 40 000 years ago, but are utterly useless to deal with today's aggravations.

Furthermore, stress today is probably more constant than it once was. In our prehistoric days, the threat of physical danger would usually pass quickly, so our systems could return to normal. However in today's fast-paced, ever changing, sue-or-be sued society, stress situations attack us virtually every waking moment. Our bodies live with a constant, low-grade fight-or-flight response, which gradually degrades our mental and physical well being.

Not only that, but we now tend to have more time to sit around and brood over our worries, mentally exaggerating minor troubles into major catastrophes. Sometimes, particularly if we are tired or upset, we can create a new problem out of the most trivial inconvenience.

Not only that, but we humans are so clever that we worry about things in advance. Our primitive ancestors – including our four-legged ones - would not have worried about next year's interest rates, or whether they were going to become redundant in the corporate downsizing next September. In other words, we now have stressors that are mainly psychological, as well as the physical, external stress agents of the world we live in.

Unfortunately your mind cannot distinguish between real physical stress and one that you are imagining. It stimulates virtually the same fight-or-flight response to an irritating on-hold telephone answering machine as it would were you fleeing from a hungry pride of lions.

The fight-or-flight response is, in short, the *physical manifestation of stress*. Every time you are stressed – and remember, for many people this is a constant, background state of being – your body maintains an active fight-or-flight response. Let's now look at how this fight-or-flight state can cause pain and other physical symptoms.

Physical health problems caused by the fight-or-flight reaction

I'm sure that you're aware that when you are stressed, your heart beats more strongly, and at a quicker rate. When this extra demand is maintained for years and decades on end, the heart's arteries can develop a series of microscopic tears. This damage encourages the formation of life-threatening clots, heightening the probability of a heart attack, or causing the pain of angina.

Not only does stress cause your heart rate to increase, but it raises your blood pressure as well. Your body initiates this reaction in an attempt to quickly deliver more blood to your extremities. Elevated blood pressure is fine during a short burst of physical exertion, but causes problems from headaches to strokes to kidney problems when maintained for too long.

Food digestion is a task far better suited to a lazy afternoon nap than the heat of a ferocious battle. It's far less important to digest your lunch than it is to avoid becoming someone else's lunch! As you would expect, the fight-or-flight response directs your body's blood flow to your muscles rather than your stomach, and slows the general activity of your digestive tract. Guess what happens if this state is maintained for too long, or is regularly repeated? That's right … tummy problems. So I hope you can see that indigestion, dyspepsia, constipation and diarrhoea are common symptoms of the anxious mind.

Stress also precipitates other changes in your blood that can cause significant health problems. For example, it causes a dramatic rise in your level of blood cholesterol and glycogen – changes that are useful in supplying energy to hard-working muscles. However, the most likely result of extra blood cholesterol and sugar these days is to predispose you to a blocked arteries or diabetes respectively.

Not only does stress heighten the activity of many organs, but, in an effort to conserve energy, it also shuts others down. All long term projects such as growth, reproduction and immunity are severely compromised by the fight-or-flight response. Hence excessive stress can cause a huge variety of seemingly unrelated health problems. For example, your bones might become weaker, leading to osteoporosis and possible fractures. Your sexual function can decrease. In yet another example, your lowered immunity means that you might become sick more often than you should.

Furthermore, constant, low-grade stress will increase the amount of hydrocortisone in your bloodstream. This hormone, which is a signature of the fight-or-flight response, has far reaching side effects. Modern medicine has simulated this hormone in a medicine called *prednisone*. It is a powerful drug that has many useful properties that help people through medical emergencies. However, this drug has tremendous side effects when taken over a prolonged period. These side effects include fluid retention, stomach ulcers, decreased immunity and brittle skin and bones.

When you are stressed, you are effectively giving yourself a small dose of this medicine. This is fine – for a while. However, if you are constantly or repeatedly stressed, the hydrocortisone in your system will slowly but surely wreak havoc with your body.

Are you starting to see the huge range of symptoms and health problems that are caused or worsened by stress? I could keep going for pages, for nearly every system has the potential to be unduly affected by prolonged stress. The two lists at the start of this chapter provide a further indication of the widespread, real, and sometimes serious consequences of prolonged stress.

In short, the fight-or-flight response forces most organs and systems to do only half their job. It shuts down the systems that are involved in long-term growth and maintenance, and overworks others involved in fighting or fleeing. If these states are maintained for too long or repeated too frequently, then something is bound to break down.

Stress and musculo-skeletal pain

Many people are interested in how stress creates musculo-skeletal problems such as neck pain, back pain, arthritis and headaches. The most common question is "how could stress possibly cause my bones and joints to degenerate?"

The process by which mental stress affects the health of your joints is somewhat complex. However, it is such and important factor in the lives of so many people that it is worth investigating in detail. About 85% of people seek treatment for these types of pains at some stage during their lives, and my guess is that many of those pains are caused, at least in part, by stress.

Your bones and joints are not under the *direct* control of your brain. The only part of your movement system that your brain directly controls is your muscles. Therefore, to understand how stress makes your bones and joints degenerate, you must first understand how your muscles control your joints.

Your body uses two different muscular systems. One group of muscles is called the *mobilising* muscles, while the other group are the *stability* muscles.

Mobilising muscles are, as their name suggests, the muscles that normally *move* your joints. Your biceps muscle in your upper arm is an example: when your contract your biceps, your elbow bends.

The mobilising muscles score all of the exciting jobs, like serving a tennis ball, drinking from a can of beer, dancing a foxtrot, or pedalling a bicycle. In general, they function when you consciously call upon them, then act in one quick burst, then rest and restore their energy.

Conversely, the stabilising muscles have the job of holding your body together, which they do in two related ways. First, they maintain your body's posture or position, such as sitting or standing. Second, the stabilising muscles counter the force of your mobilising muscles during joint movement. Without the stabilising muscles, your mobilising muscles would probably pull your joints out of place!

Your mind subconsciously recruits your stability muscles for all the tedious, boring jobs, such as posture maintenance, joint stability, and holding your organs in place. Because of this requirement, your stability muscles function with a continuous, low intensity contraction, and you are usually barely aware that they are working.

Sometimes, your stabilising muscles become weak, while your mobilising muscles grow stronger. This imbalance between the two sets of muscles means that your bones do not glide properly along each other when you move a joint. The resulting uncontrolled movement makes the joint or adjacent tendons degenerate very quickly.

This effect can be likened a car tyre: if the wheels are properly balanced and aligned then the tyre will wear evenly across its surface, and will last for years. However, if the wheels are badly aligned or unbalanced, one side of the tyre will wear out far more quickly.

Your joints are the same. An unbalanced movement pattern creates extra wear-and-tear, meaning that you will injure yourself more frequently, more easily, or that your injuries will be more difficult to cure. If this wear-and-tear is left unchecked for many years, then osteoarthritis, tendonitis, muscle knots or spinal pain may develop.

As such, the balance between your stabilising muscles and your mobilising muscles is one of the most important aspects of joint health.

Without this balance, you are far more likely to injure yourself, and you will be especially prone to developing wear-and-tear type injuries.

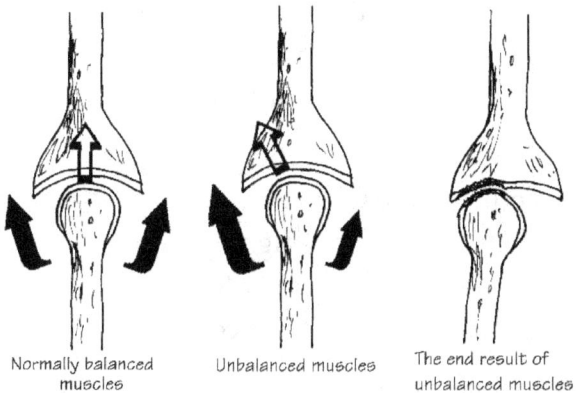

Normally balanced muscles · Unbalanced muscles · The end result of unbalanced muscles

How does all of this apply to the effects of stress? Here's my theory.

Let's again consider the fight-or-flight response. If you were about to be speared through the buttocks by the horn of a raging *Triceratops* dinosaur, which group of muscles would you rather have ready to fire? Would you rather that your body used:

> (a) the stabilising muscles, which securely hold the joints in a correct position, and maintain a good posture, or

(b) the mobilising muscles, which will help you to run away?

If you said 'a' then you would have made a very nice entree for the triceratops. However, if you thought that the mobilising muscles would be more useful in this situation, then I congratulate you for a correct response.

Can you guess what happens to your mobilising muscles if you are constantly tense and anxious? That's right, your body holds them on full alert, ready to produce fight-or-flight at a moment's notice.

Many people carry excess stress in their mobilising muscles. Hunching, tight neck and shoulder muscles are a common example. Another frequently observed example are the jaw muscles, which, as any dentist can tell you, often become tight, causing nocturnal teeth-grinding (providing yet another holiday in the Whitsunday Islands for the dentist).

If the mobilising muscles are frequently or constantly held in this highly reactive state, they gradually develop extra tone and strength. Meanwhile, the stabilising muscles lie relatively quietly. After some time, the two muscle groups develop an imbalance. You know what happens next: the muscle imbalance causes degeneration in nearby joints, eventually leading to pain and injury. *Voila*, your stress has caused joint degeneration, injury or arthritis. And, unfortunately, chronic pain!

Stress increases your perception of pain

Another way that chronic, low-grade stress creates extra problems is by heightening your *perception* of pain.[*] Small irritations can become noticeable, while moderate pains can be made to feel intolerable. For example, consider a low-grade headache, which seems to throb with extra intensity when you are upset.

This difference in perceived pain occurs even though the physical pain signals arising from your body are identical. In other words, *the*

---

[*] As an interesting side note, extreme stress can actually diminish pain by causing the body to release morphine-like chemicals into the bloodstream. However, this stress-induced analgesia is usually confined to extreme situations such as the battlefield or sports ground, so we won't discuss it any further.

same amount of pain hurts more when you are stressed rather than relaxed.

This effect works in reverse as well. A calm, peaceful mind perceives less pain than does an active mind. Some people - Himalayan yogis, for example - can meditate and relax so deeply that they feel no pain at all. As one Yogi said with complete seriousness: 'I feel pain ... but it does not hurt.' Wouldn't that be nice!

Deep hypnotherapy can produce the same results, and can be so effective that deeply relaxed, hypnotised people have undergone surgery without anaesthetic.

Obviously, your state of mind can alter your pain perception. To understand how this effect occurs, you must appreciate a simple mechanism known as the *gate theory* of pain.

When a structure in your body such as a joint, muscle or ligament is injured, it sends pain messages up certain fibres of the nearby nerves. These signals then enter into your spinal cord, through which they travel up to the brain. When the message enters the spinal cord, it must cross over a small joint, known as a *synapse*. Think of a synapse as being like an electrical switch that joins two wires together and you get a rough picture.

The relationship between the spinal cord nerves and the peripheral nerves is not necessarily one-to-one. The synapse area in the spinal cord has the ability to allow many, just a few, or almost none of these incoming messages up the spinal cord. Of course, if the signals cannot pass up the spinal cord, then they do not register in the brain as pain.

The spinal cord acts like a gate - hence the name 'gate theory' - in allowing only a varied number of signals up at a time. In effect, the spinal cord has the capability to control how many pain sensations you are experiencing, which of course dictates your level of discomfort.

How does the gate theory relate stress to pain? It is likely that stress opens more gates in your spinal cord. In prehistoric days this response would have been useful, priming the spinal cord to receive signals from the limbs. In this way, your ancestor's reactions would have been very responsive and sensitive - useful qualities in a dangerous situation.

You have probably noticed that your nerves become 'edgy' when you are tense, and that you become overly responsive to stimulation that would not normally affect you. For example, if you are stressed and someone claps his or her hands, you startle. However, if this same noise occurred when you were relaxed, you would barely notice it. This hypersensitivity is a simple example of how the flight-or-fight response primes your nerves to receive even the smallest signals.

If you are stressed, the fight-or-flight response opens many spinal cord gates, meaning that more of the pain messages ascend to your brain. In this way, stress can cause minor pain to feel awful, and an otherwise bearable injury can become intolerable.

Sometimes a vicious cycle can develop, in which your pain causes you to feel stressed, which increases your perception of the pain. Naturally, the extra discomfort makes you even more anxious, which further heightens your pain, and so on.

However, the gate theory of pain is not all bad news. If you can learn to deeply relax, your brain will close the gates in the spinal cord. Why should it waste time and energy monitoring your limbs when you are not in any danger? The end result: you feel less pain.

In this chapter, you learned...

I hope that you can now see that stress not only causes emotional changes such as irritability and short temperedness, but can also create a whole range of physical problems. Many diseases, even those with measurable, identifiable causes, are precipitated or worsened by the fight-or-flight response. Not only that, but chronic stress can lead to physical injury, and heightens your perception of pain.

It follows that to decrease your pain and illness, you have to learn to control the fight-or-flight responses that are occurring within your own body. Soon, you will learn techniques that will help you to master this important method of self control.

Let's now look at another important area: your *physical tolerance to stress*. The next chapter will show you in simple terms how your stress level and your physical tolerance to stress affect your health.

Chapter Three
"Your physical tolerance to stress"

Why some people are always sick,
while others are usually healthy

Your physical tolerance to stress

Ill health and well being seem to affect people in a vastly disproportionate manner. For example, you probably know a few 'hypochondriacs' who are always sore or sick. They're always suffering with a cough or cold, their back is constantly sore, and they visit a health practitioner virtually every week. Even worse, they regularly provide you with an avalanche of unrequested details about their numerous maladies.

Equally, I'm sure that you've also met people who rarely have any aches or pains, and never catch any bugs that are going around. Are these people just lucky?

Between these two extremes are a vast majority of people, who have occasional problems, and intermittent aches and pains.

(Ask yourself now: to which group do *you* belong?)

Why does health vary so much from one person to the next, even though we are all subject to similar everyday hazards? The answer may well lie in how we physically tolerate stress.

Consider the following graphs. Suppose that the dotted line represents your *stress level*. As you'd expect, it goes up and down in response to life's challenges. Sometimes things are going well, and stress is minimal. Other times, life doesn't seem as easy, and your anxiety increases. As you'd expect, the dotted line on the following graphs naturally oscillates, just as does the stress of life.

The solid line represents your *physical tolerance to stress*. This line represents your body's constitution. It is influenced by factors such as diet, exercise, disease and sleep.

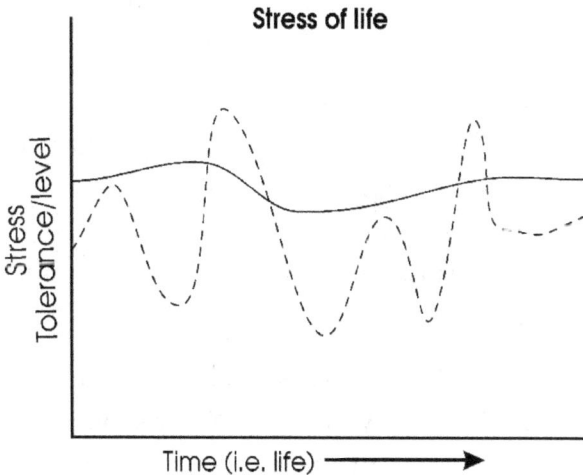

Stress of life

Stress Tolerance/level

Time (i.e. life) ⟶

The height of this line represents the amount of stress that your body can physically handle before it breaks down. When you are sleeping soundly, eating sensibly and exercising regularly, your physical tolerance to stress rises. If you skip meals, work too hard or drink too little, er, sorry, I meant drink too much, your physical tolerance may fall. As you'd expect, this line also creeps slowly up and down.

When the dotted stress level is above the solid line of your physical stress tolerance, injury, pain or illnesses are imminent. At times such as this, your mind and body simply cannot cope with the degree of stress to which you are subjecting them. Something *must* give.

This breakdown does not necessarily happen straight away. While there are many recorded instances of stress precipitating a sudden severe reaction such as a heart attack or stroke, most problems are caused by chronic, low-grade, constant stress.

Living with chronic stress can be likened to forgetting to clean your teeth every day. If you don't clean your teeth for one or two nights, you won't instantly develop a cavity.

However, if you regularly ignore dental hygiene for years, you will not only lose most of your friends, but most of your teeth as well.

Similarly, one or two stressful incidents will normally do you no harm whatsoever. The fight-or-flight response is designed for such situations. However, if you constantly or regularly stress yourself beyond the capacity of your body to cope, then you will eventually pay the price.

As shown in the last chapter, your body has a variety of ways of pointing this out to you, including physical problems, mental disorders, and, of course, pain. Let's look at some fictitious cases - we'll use three of the seven dwarfs - and see in general terms how our bodies react to excessive stress, and to the general way that we are treating them.

First, consider the case of 'Happy', who we'll represent in graph one. Happy has a very high stress tolerance, and a very low stress level. Even during periods of high anxiety, her body and mind remain within their capacity to cope. Consequently, Happy is almost never sick, has no chronic pain, and comfortably copes with her lot in life.

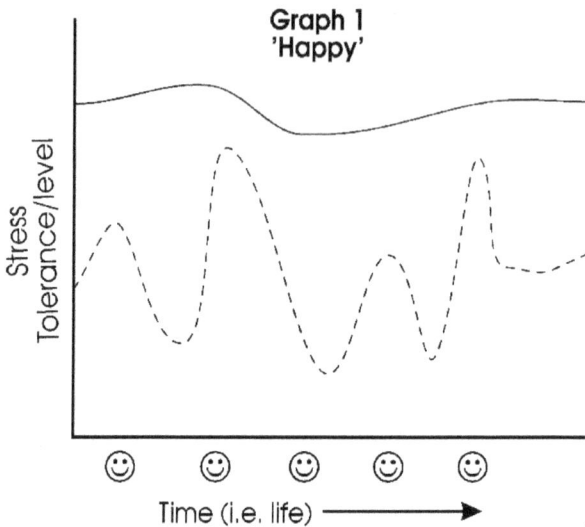

Graph 1
'Happy'

Stress Tolerance/level

Time (i.e. life) ⟶

Graph two represents another person/dwarf, 'Grumpy'. Grumpy's stress level is typically very high, while his stress tolerance is unfortunately very low. As a result, Grumpy's body and mind are in a constant state of disrepair. He drinks alcohol excessively, is often sick, suffers frequent bouts of depression, and has a long-standing skin rash. Grumpy has also suffered with a chronic, generalised backache for ten years, which he blames on his job.

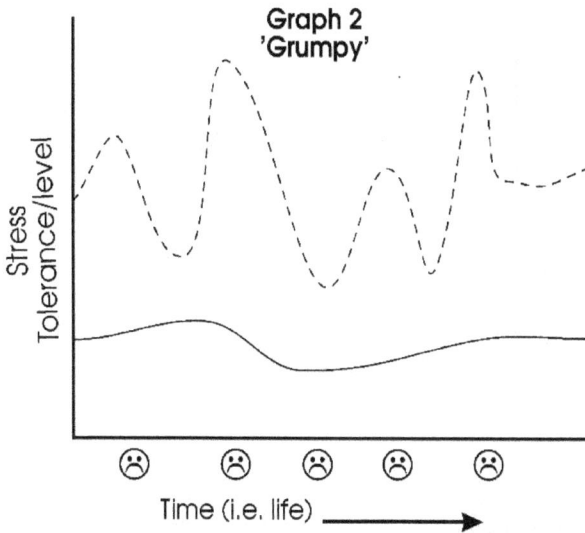

Graph 2
'Grumpy'

Stress
Tolerance/level

Time (i.e. life)

Obviously, both Happy and Grumpy are extreme examples, although Grumpy's case may be more common than you realise. Other people may be more closely represented by the dwarf in graph three, which we'll call 'Doc'. Doc's stress tolerance is fairly steady, but, like most of us, his stress level fluctuates from month to month. During the periods in which Doc's stress level rises above the capacity of his body to cope, something collapses.

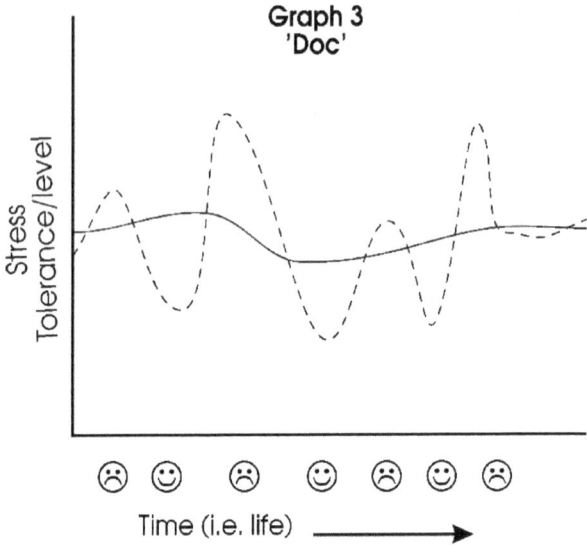

Graph 3
'Doc'

Stress Tolerance/level

Time (i.e. life)

Therefore, Doc occasionally feels nauseous, and he has headaches from time to time. Sometimes, he simply has no energy. Yet rarely does he associate any of his symptoms directly with stress. Instead he blames other more tangible factors for his problems, such as the weather, food poisoning, the wicked witch, or any one of a thousand other causes of minor maladies.

Now, let's look at how these situations can change. Let's suppose that - as shown in graph four - Doc increases his stress tolerance. Now, even during stressful times, his body is able to cope without breaking down.

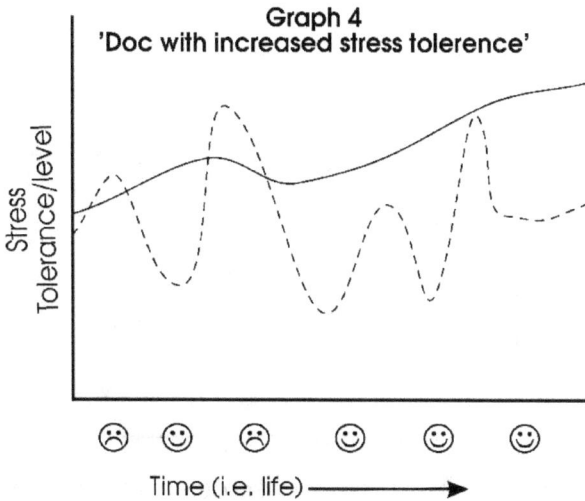

Graph 4
'Doc with increased stress tolerence'

The same effect occurs if Doc lowers his stress level, as shown in graph five. Again, his body rarely reaches the point of breakdown, and as such he is happier and healthier. Funnily, his headaches seem remarkably good during these times, which he attributes to a magic potion that his fairy godmother brewed last summer.

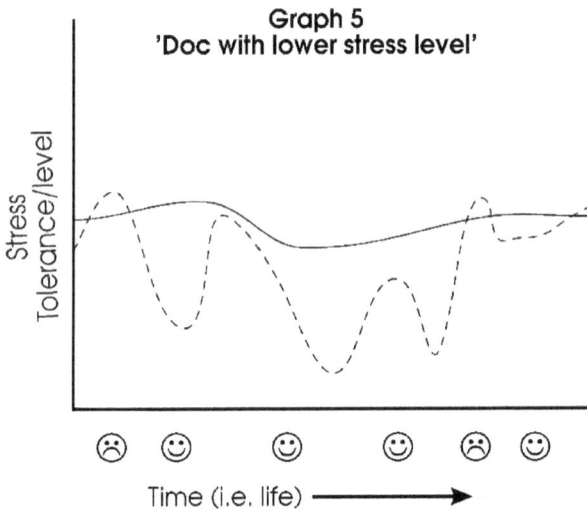

Graph 5
'Doc with lower stress level'

Stress Tolerance/level

Time (i.e. life) ⟶

Naturally, these affects also occur in reverse. For example, consider Happy again, and suppose that her physical stress tolerance decreases, as in graph six, or her stress level increases, as in graph seven. In either of these situations, Happy will feel the physical and mental detriments of stress. She will become sick, emotionally unstable, or maybe develop bodily aches and pains.

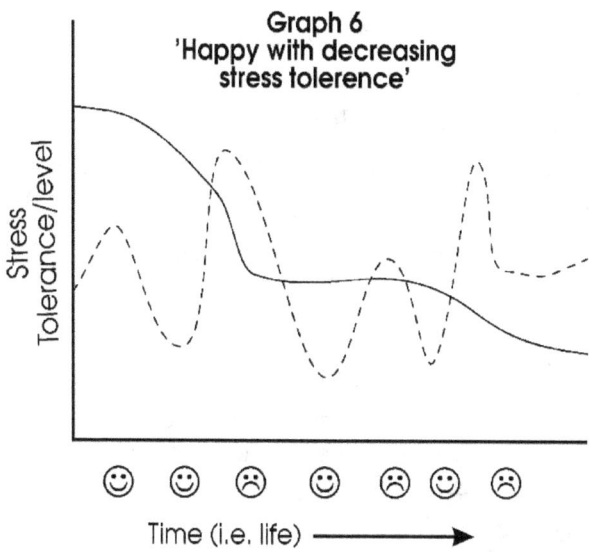

Graph 6
'Happy with decreasing stress tolerence'

Stress Tolerance/level

☺ ☺ ☹ ☺ ☹ ☺ ☹

Time (i.e. life) ⟶

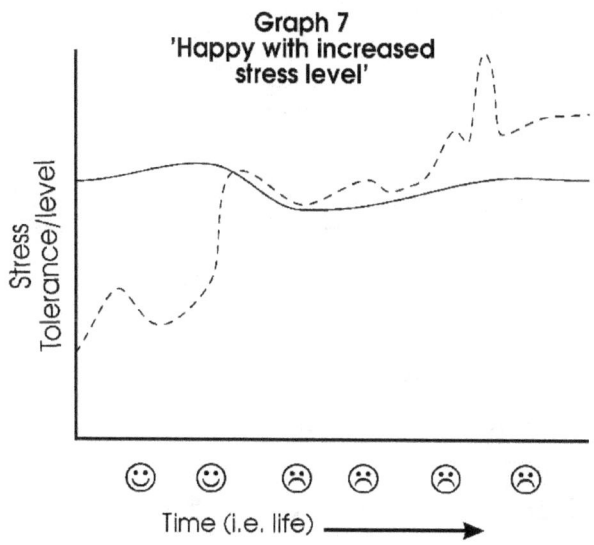

Graph 7
'Happy with increased stress level'

Stress Tolerance/level

☺ ☺ ☹ ☹ ☹ ☹

Time (i.e. life) ⟶

Finally, back to poor old Grumpy. Grumpy's best hope is to decrease his stress level *and* increase his stress tolerance, as shown in graph eight. Not an impossible task, but he's going to require a lot of dedication and persistence to work his way out of his present situation.

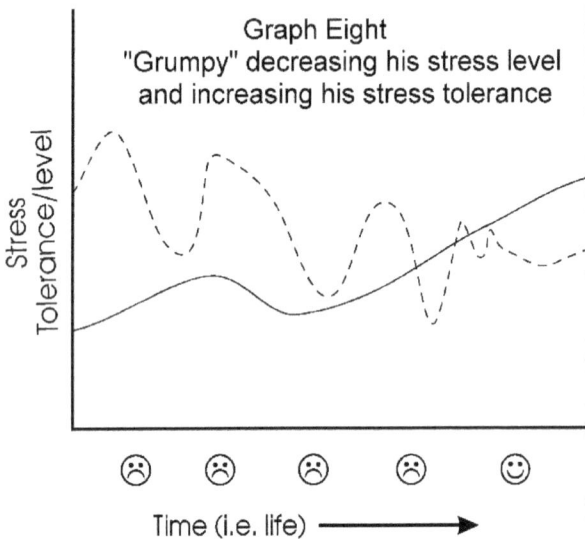

Graph Eight
"Grumpy" decreasing his stress level and increasing his stress tolerance

Stress Tolerance/level

Time (i.e. life) ⟶

Can you see that although life still has its difficulties, stress doesn't have to affect us? By learning to either decrease your stress level, or increase your tolerance to stress, you can create a situation in which you can cope, no matter what life throws at you.

How do we take these two important steps? Let's find out.

Increasing your physical tolerance to stress

The secret to increasing your physical tolerance to stress can be summarised in one sentence.

Listen to your mother.

That's right, just do all those things that your mother always told you to do: eat properly, get plenty of sleep, exercise regularly, blah blah blah. (Of course, if your mother regularly advised you to take up heroin, then you should probably ignore her.)

But seriously, most people are aware of the rules for healthy living: eat plenty of fresh fruit and vegies, sleep for about eight hours per night, drink lots of water, and perform thirty minutes of solid exercise four times per week.

Yet despite these simple, undeniable, self-evident rules for a happy, healthy, stress-free lifestyle, many people ignore them. The media is crammed with fad diets, crazy nutritional supplements and totally inappropriate 'fat burning' exercise gadgets that would be laughable were they not so popular.

It is beyond the scope of this booklet to discuss these topics in greater detail. Your local library is brimming with thousands of publications that will guide you further in these areas. *Back pain: How to get Rid of it Forever*, by this author, contains further commonsense advice on areas such as diet, exercise, medication, strengthening and stretching.

In short, I'm sure that you already know the rules of healthy living. I hope you have already integrated into your life. If not, then this booklet will help you to develop the mindset to do so.

Decreasing your stress level

You have two techniques available to help you to decrease your stress level.

First, you could change the things that stress you. The other technique is to change yourself, so that external situations and happenings do not make you as stressed. Here, an old saying springs to mind.

> *(Lord, Budda, Allah, Ghost who walks, God ... insert the deity of your choice)*
> *Grant me the serenity to accept the things that I cannot change*
> *The courage to change the things that I can*
> *And the wisdom to know the difference.*

Which method is best for you? Let's first look at some common situations that cause stress. This will help you to decide if they are changeable. Some common causes of stress include the following internal and external factors:

(a) Your personality type.

Research has shown that certain personality types are likely to suffer from stress. These people, known to psychologists as Type A personalities, tend to push themselves hard, be rarely satisfied with their own performance, are hostile in traffic, and are intolerant of other people. Ring any bells? Cynical, mistrusting people are also very prone to high stress levels.

(b) Repressed anger.

Are you carrying a deep grudge against someone who offended your self-esteem at some stage - a divorced partner, or an ex-boss, for example? Repressed anger has been shown to be a major stress agent, particularly in men.

(c) Guilt.

People develop guilt about a whole range of issues: eating too much, sexual guilt, guilt because of early childhood experiences, just to name a few. Women tend to be vulnerable to guilt-related stress.

(d) Negative self-talk.

Any time you rethink negative thoughts, your stress level will naturally rise. People who tend to brood, sulk or feel resentful are particularly prone to this type of stress, as are people who are naturally pessimistic.

(e) Wrong job.

A job that you dislike, or that does not suit your natural strengths and weaknesses, can be a major cause of stress.

(f) Change.

A new job, a relationship separation, moving house, even a new car ... anything that represents a change also represents a stress factor. Modern life and technology is not only changing more quickly than ever before, but the rate of change is accelerating. No wonder we're all so stressed.

Excessive or major change is such an important contributor to stress that psychologists have developed charts for measuring the amount of change in your life. Major events, such as the death of a spouse, are assigned very high points, while other changes such as moving house are assigned fewer points. Your score on this 'life change scale' has been experimentally shown to accurately predict your general level of health over the ensuing year.

(g) Lack of control

Experiments on animals suggest that having control of your life is very important to mediate stress. For example, rats who were trained to push a lever when they wanted food were found to have lower stress levels than those who received an identical amount of food, but at random intervals during the day.

(h) Lack of predictability

Animal studies have also shown that a certain amount of predictability also aids stress reduction. In one study, one group of rats was administered a stress-inducing series of tiny electric shocks[*]. A second group of rats received a similar series of shocks, but received a warning bell a few seconds before the shock was delivered. This group developed far less stress-related illness did the first group.

Why? Well, it's difficult to ask a rat, but the researchers suspect that the forewarned rats were more able to relax for the rest of the time, thus decreasing their overall anxiety.

---

[*] By the way, the shocks were only tiny. While modern medicine avoids animal experiments where possible, stress research is not readily carried out by examining a test tube.

However, the rats in the first group were constantly on guard, never knowing when the zap would hit next. They concluded that, in some human situations, the same stress agent will have less negative effects if you are forewarned.

(i) No physical outlet for frustrations

Having a physical outlet for your frustration has been shown experimentally to decrease stress. One interesting project studied the stress hormone levels in male baboons who have just lost a fight with another baboon – quite a stressful experience for a young, up-and-coming baboon with an eye for the leadership of the group. They found that the losing baboons had lower stress responses if they physically express their anger rather than bottling it up.

For we humans, sport and exercise fills a wonderful role in this regard.

As an interesting side note, some companies in Japan supply a dummy that looks like the boss on which employees can physically vent their frustrations. Apparently, these workplaces are more harmonious and calm.

Depending on what you think of your boss, this revelation may or may not surprise you.

(j) Lack of social support

Health benefits of many kinds can be derived from having a good network of family and friends. Some studies even report lower levels of stress hormones in people who own a pet!

(k) Anything else that you can think of.

You're partner, co-workers, traffic, your children, your parents, money, that leaking tap, lack of time, too much time ... I could go on for pages. So far, I've barely scratched the surface.

Are you starting to see how many causes of stress may be in your life? Are you going to change them all?

Not likely.

Sure, you may be able to alter some of the major causes of stress in your life, using the above list as a starting point. Change jobs, for example, or join a new sporting club. Furthermore, working on your own attitudes - such as decreasing your resentment toward other people who have wronged you - can produce major benefits in stress reduction.

However, it is extremely unlikely that the world is going to slow down for a couple of months, just so that little old you and I can take a breather.

Some people take this approach to an extreme: they resign from their jobs, and move to a self sustaining farm in the hills, content to live out their days doing nothing but ambling through the woods, recording their thoughts in a journal. Sure, it's good work if you can get it, but I'd guess that this solution is not going to suit most people.

Common sense will tell you that many of the stress agents in your life are outside your bounds of influence, and therefore you cannot change them.

So what should you do? Simply, you learn to accept those things that would formerly have distressed you, and to reduce the manifestations of any stress that you may experience.

In short, you have to do what Doc did in graph five: lower the dotted line that represents your stress level. The easiest way to do this is to learn *deep relaxation of your mind*. In the next chapter, we'll examine in detail how to achieve this peace-of-mind, and the benefits that come with it.

Chapter Four
"How to relax"

Eat more cake and drink more beer?

Exercises to decrease stress

'I know how to relax. It's easy. I just grab a six pack out of the fridge, lie on the couch, and watch sport on television all day.'

'If I want to relax, I just drop the kids off at Mum's place, then call a girlfriend to go out for coffee and a huge slice of mud cake.'

Sorry. Relaxation is not that simple.

Sure, the alcohol or chocolate may temporarily make you feel better. Moreover, for many men, doing something simple like watching sport is a simple way to forget problems, while many women find that a good chat will help them resolve their difficulties. Although you may find these activities enjoyable, they unfortunately don't produce the deep mental relaxation that you need to rid yourself of stress and its associated pains and problems.

The colloquial use of the word 'relaxation' differs from the concept to which we are referring. Here, the term 'relaxation' does not mean eating, drinking and being merry, but rather refers to the practice of deeply calming your state of mind. From now on, if I use the term 'relaxed' I am referring to a state of *deep mental relaxation,* NOT to how you feel when you are having fun.

What exactly is a *deeply relaxed mind,* and how does it differ from your normal state? A deeply relaxed mind is a floating, uncritical mind, which thinks its own thoughts. If your mind is deeply relaxed, you do not analyse, worry, or direct your thinking in any way. Your mental processes have no logic, and you do not attempt to understand, resolve or clarify any thoughts that enter your head.

You may be vaguely familiar with this state if you've ever found yourself daydreaming. When you daydream, your mind drifts along without obvious direction. You are oblivious to your surroundings, and uncritical of anything that occurs nearby. The moment of reverie just before you fall asleep provides another close approximation.

When you're doing the relaxation exercises, you must learn to let yourself go to this deeply relaxed, floating, drifting state of mind.

You will soon be learning how to perform relaxation exercises. The exercises have four main benefits.

1.   You will learn how to relax your muscles, easing any tension or tightness.

2.   Your relaxed state of mind will diminish your pain perception.[*]

3.   The calm and peaceful feeling will stay with you after you have finished the exercises, promoting general well being.

4.   When your mind is deeply relaxed, you can use various other techniques to alter how you think about your pain.

Let's now look at some practical tips on how to best perform these extremely useful exercises.

Some practical considerations for performing the relaxation exercises

---

[*] As mentioned at the start of this booklet, deep mental relaxation should never be used to repress pain of unknown origin. The techniques can be so powerful that even very dangerous pain can be masked. Use your common sense, and consult an appropriate health practitioner if you are unsure.

Do not be put off by their simplicity

Because of the deeply relaxed state of mind that the following exercises engender, the instructions that you give to yourself are, by nature, very simple. Your mind, in its current active state, will probably perceive the instructions as so straightforward as to be almost useless. Do not be put off by this simplicity!

Complicated sentences or detailed instructions would not be as readily accepted by your relaxed mind as simple, direct statements. As you progress through the exercises, your mind will gradually let go, and the simple statements will have a deep impact on your way of thinking.

Practice makes perfect

Don't worry if at first you have difficulty in achieving a fully relaxed state. These mental routines are like any other skill: they take time, practice and persistence to learn properly. Very few people would expect to pick up a golf club for the first time and hit a perfect drive. Skills such as this take training and practice to master. Most of my mates have been playing golf for fifteen years and are still no closer to having a decent swing.

Similarly, deep mental relaxation is a skill that is not self-evident, but must be learned. Don't be surprised if your first few efforts are not a spectacular success. Frequently, beginners have trouble with random thoughts and worries interrupting the flow of the exercises. If this happens, simply 'let the thought go', and gently redirect your attention back to the exercise phrases. I'm sure with a little practice that you'll start to experience that calm, floating feeling, and will soon discover how natural and peaceful it is to relax.

It gets quicker

You will find that when you master the skills of relaxation, you will be able to achieve a calm, peaceful mind far more quickly than in your first attempts. During the first few weeks that you attempt these exercises, you may find that it takes half an hour or more to achieve a deeply relaxed state. After a few months of practice, most people can achieve deep relaxation within five or ten minutes.

I have seen experiments in which highly practiced subjects were able to block out all pain signals after only twenty seconds of relaxation. They proved their immunity to pain by keeping their hands in a bath of icy water for two minutes, without any increase in pain level, heart rate or respiration. I wouldn't advise you to try that experiment at home, but if you've ever fished through the bottom of an ice-filled esky, searching for the last cold stubby, then I'm sure you can appreciate how deeply relaxed these subjects must have been. And they could achieve this painless state of mind in just twenty seconds!

Not only that, but as you improve your mental relaxation skills, you will find that the feeling of calm stays with you for longer periods. Many people who are experienced in these techniques find that they require only a few minutes of relaxation to maintain an all-day feeling of calm and peacefulness. Not a bad pay off for five minutes effort. Don't you agree?

Be alert and awake when you perform the exercises

Many people believe that when you sleep that your mind is completely relaxed. This assumption is not necessarily true. Many people sleep fitfully, tossing and turning ideas through their mind all night. Others find that each time they awaken, a problem is churning away in their semi-conscious mind. Many people take drugs or alcohol in order to sleep, both of which promote a false sense of relaxation.

Compare these states to a floating, calm, peaceful mind as described above, and you will see that sleep does not necessarily provide deep relaxation.

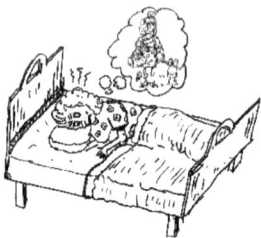

For this reason, you should perform these exercises when you are alert and fully awake. Otherwise, you may nod off to sleep before you have achieved a fully relaxed state, and you won't achieve the benefits for your mind or body that it can bring.

Later, when you have mastered the exercises and have reaped the benefits of a relaxed mind, you may wish to use the exercises to help you fall asleep at night. However, I suggest that you avoid this practice for at least six weeks, in order that you make the fastest possible progress with the development of your new skill.

Use a posture that is slightly uncomfortable

Most people naturally presume that a warm, cosy, comfortable position will assist with mental relaxation. In fact, the opposite is more likely to be true: a slightly uncomfortable posture will help you attain a more deeply relaxed mental state.

An overly comfortable posture can trick your brain into thinking that you are relaxed. By keeping your body slightly inconvenienced, your mind will realise that it has not yet achieved a fully relaxed state, and will continue to allow your muscles and mind to let go.

Picture a Buddhist monk, or a Himalyan yogi, deep in meditation. How do you think they would position themselves? On the couch? In a hammock? On a soft, feathery bed? Not likely. Most people who are adept at deep relaxation sit on a hard floor, often in a crossed-legged position. In this 'lotus' position, the meditating person can pull their feet further underneath them as they reach progressively deeper states of relaxation. This action creates extra tension and mild discomfort in the legs, thus inviting the mind to relax even more deeply.

This principal is useful for you, too, although you may not wish to take it as far as the lotus position. Just make sure that you are not too comfortable, and you'll be fine.

What posture is best for the exercises?

The easiest position to try is sitting. Just ensure that your chair is supportive yet not too heavily padded. Your feet should be resting flat on the floor, with your hands on the armrests or in your lap. Your head may drop forward onto your chest as you relax more deeply.

Alternatively, you may be more comfortable in a lying posture, possibly with a pillow under your knees. Here, I recommend that you lie on a firm surface such as the floor, rather than a soft, comfortable bed. You may use a small pillow or, preferably, a folded towel under your head if necessary.

The ideal posture for you depends upon many factors, such as the time and place that you have put aside in which to perform your relaxation exercises. In general, any posture will do, so long as it is not too comfortable.

Some other general hints for posture are:
- Keep your limbs symmetrical
- Minimise or loosen your clothing
- Keep your arms and legs uncrossed

Where to do the exercises

In the beginning, you should choose a place in which you feel totally safe and secure. Have your back or head nearest to the wall, which will provide you with an extra feeling of safety. Take the telephone off the hook, and put up a physical or otherwise tangible 'do not disturb' sign. The light should be dim but not dark, and the room should be relatively quiet. These provisions will allow you to more easily slip into an unguarded, relaxed state of mind.

As you improve your relaxation skills, you should move out of your comfort zone. Progress through steps such as trying the exercises with the radio or television turned on. In this way, you will learn to tolerate and relax against background noise. You may wish to try the exercises in a more uncomfortable location - one expert used to lie on a rocky stone wall in his garden - or with your eyes open. By increasing the uncomfortableness of your surrounds, you will teach your mind to relax in a variety of circumstances.

After a few months practice, you will be ready to attempt the exercises in the arena of real life. People skilled in these techniques can attain a deeply relaxed state in almost any situation, from a crowded bus to walking down the city street. Athletes such as swimmers and runners may even wish to try the mental exercises when training. Many great athletes have even used them in the midst of competition!

Finally, you can use the techniques in known stressful situations. Imagine how useful your relaxation skills would be before your next big job interview or after-dinner speech. Of course, these techniques, once mastered, will prove invaluable when you are suffering from acute or chronic pain.

A word of common sense: don't try these exercises while driving home from work, or while operating the backhoe that you've hired for the weekend from the hardware store. Obviously, a floating, uncritical mind is not an appropriate state in which to attempt dangerous, reactive or mentally challenging tasks.

Really 'feel' the instructions

The relaxation exercises are represented by a series of phrases that you say to yourself. However, just repeating the statements to yourself does not necessarily ensure that your mind will follow the instructions. You must really try to 'feel' the instructions, and allow your mind to follow as they suggest.

This practice of *allowing* your mind to feel the instructions - rather than forcing it to follow them - is one of the keys to obtaining a deeply relaxed mental state. Again, this method of thinking requires practice, but will come soon enough if you persist, relax, and keep gently reminding yourself of its importance.

Learn how to let go of physical tension

Some people find it very difficult to fully let go of physical tension in the muscles. To discover if you are one of these people, try this simple test.

Have someone else lift your arm into the air, and hold it for a few seconds. Then, without warning, they should suddenly release your arm. Observe what happens. If your arm naturally flops to your side without resistance - it should drop with a completely passive flop, not an active, pulling down movement - then you are probably fairly physically relaxed.

However, you may find that your arm hovers in the air for a fraction of a second, indicating moderately high stress levels. Some people are so physically tense that they are unable to let their arm fall at all, instead just deliberately lowering it to a resting position.

Letting go of muscle tension is simple but vital skill that you must learn. To be able to let go of muscle tone, you must first learn to identify it. Following is a simple task that will teach you the simple skill of identifying increased muscle tone.

Sit or lie comfortably. Now concentrate on your right thigh. Feel, and try to really experience, how much tone and tension are in the muscle.

Next, pretend to lift your right leg. Don't actually move it, but simply pretend that you are about to, so that its weight on the bed or chair is minimal. Do you sense the increased tension in the front thigh muscle?

The state in which you are now holding your right thigh muscle is one of increased muscle tone. Feel and knead your thigh with your fingers, and compare its suppleness to your left thigh. You will note that the right side feels much harder, while your left thigh muscle is softer, relaxed and more pliable.

Now relax the muscle, and experience the feeling of softening, and 'letting go'. This 'letting go' feeling is very important, and forms the basis for the following exercises. Practice this action of 'letting go' once or twice more before you read on.

Try to develop a conscious awareness of muscle tone and the all-important feeling of letting go while you perform the relaxation exercises.

Don't worry if you cannot remember the instructions word-for-word

As you perform the relaxation techniques for the first couple of times, you will probably have to read the phrases from this book. This method is fine, and will help you to develop a feel for the exercises.

Alternatively, this booklet has a companion MP3 track that you can download for free. This guided relaxation session is an invaluable guide in your first few months of practice, as it will allow you to let your mind drift, without the extra burden of guiding the trains of thought. See our website www.JPpublishingAUSTRALIA.com for details.

As you become more adept, you should close your eyes and mentally repeat the instructions to yourself. Do not worry if you cannot remember the instructions perfectly. As long as you remember the general stages of the whole process, you can virtually invent your own relaxation phrases as you go.

The phrases below and on the compact disc are just examples to get you started. You may find that some ideas work for you, while others have no calming effect whatsoever. Fine. Stick with the instructions that work best for you, and disregard any that you don't find helpful.

If you create your own phrases, always use positive instructions such as 'I feel...' or 'I am...', rather than negative instructions such as 'I do not feel...' or 'I am not....' For example, use a phrase such as 'I feel calm and relaxed' rather than telling yourself 'I don't feel stressed'. You will see later why this type of positive thinking is so important.

The relaxation exercises

The relaxation exercises follow a natural, logical sequence of stages that will guide you from being alert and tense, through to being fully, deeply relaxed.

First, you will prepare your mind for the relaxation that is to follow. Then, you progressively relax each body part, using a technique known as *contract-relax*. To perform the contract-relax technique, follow these simple steps. Try it as you read, by squeezing your right hand into a fist.

(1) When you next inhale, tighten the target muscle as firmly as possible. Hold for a few seconds as you experience the tension in the muscle.

(2) Then, on your next outward breath, allow the muscle to suddenly and completely relax. Experience the feeling of letting go.

(3) Allow yourself another inward breath. Then, as you exhale, relax the same muscle even more completely. Just aim for the same 'letting go' feeling that you used in step two. Try to really feel the relaxation.

(4) When your next inward breath arrives, move on to the next muscle as described.

This routine may sound a bit complicated, but it is very simple and logical when you're used to it. In short, you tightly contract a muscle, then spend your next two exhalations relaxing it, before moving on to the next muscle group.

After physically relaxing your limbs and trunk, you should move your awareness to your face, scalp and eyes. Then allow the relaxation to permeate through to your mind. You will start to feel as though you are floating, and your thoughts will wander as you gradually slip into deep relaxation.

Once in this state of mind, you have three options, which we'll discuss later. Finally, after having worked through all the stages, you slowly and gently bring yourself back to reality, feeling calm, peaceful and pain free.

Let's now examine these steps individually, and discover the simple exercises that can make such a difference to your physical and mental well being.

By the way, the following sections won't make very interesting reading if you simply skim over them. I suggest that you try the techniques as you read. That's right ... try to feel and use the simple phrases as you go. In this way you will experience first hand just how simple and effective these techniques can be. Do it!

(1) Preparation for relaxation

Take a slow, deep breath. Let your whole body relax as you allow yourself to exhale. Do not force the breath out; simply allow it to flow out of your body, like a long sigh.

Repeat this long, relaxed sigh two more times, aiming for a relaxed, heavy, calm feeling during each exhalation.

Inwardly experience the following sentiments as you slowly, carefully repeat them to yourself. (Remember that their simplicity is a virtue that you will come to appreciate.)

> *I have nothing else to do for the next twenty minutes.*
> *This is my time to relax.*
> *I feel safe, I feel secure.*
> *I deserve to feel relaxed.*
> *It feels good to relax.*
> *I feel calm.*
> *Calm and relaxed.*

Now take another deep, relaxing breath, and move to stage two.

(2) Progressive physical relaxation

Use the following movements and phrases to guide you through a cycle of contract-relax exercises.

Turn your attention to your feet.
As you breathe in, curl your toes up tightly.
Feel the tension in the arches of your feet.
Breathe out, and relax your feet.
Let go of your feet.
Allow yourself to take another inward breath.
As you exhale, relax your feet even further.
Feel the relaxation.
It feels good to relax your feet.
Turn your attention to your calf muscles.
As you breathe in, push your toes away from you.
Feel the tension in your calf muscles.
Breathe out, and relax your calf muscles.
Let go of your calf muscles.
Allow yourself to take another inward breath.
As you exhale, relax your calf muscles even further.
Feel the relaxation.
It feels good to relax your calf muscles.

Get the picture? The process may sound repetitive, but as you try the exercises, you will see that a simple, repeatable formula is best.

As you have already relaxed your feet and calves, I suggest that you next move to your thighs. First, tighten and relax your quadriceps muscles. Then contract your hamstring muscles, which is most easily achieved by pressing your heel into the floor. Then move to your front hip muscles (pretend to lift your leg in the air) and then to your buttocks (squeeze your bottom cheeks together). Simply follow the same pattern as you did when your released your feet and calf muscles. After this, you may find it useful to let your *whole* legs go, and reaffirm your commitment to ease and calm. Try some phrases such as these:

> *My whole legs are relaxed.*
> *Utterly relaxed.*
> *Relaxed and loose.*
> *It feels good to relax my legs.*
> *My legs are so relaxed that they are heavy.*
> *I can feel the weight of my legs*
> *My legs feel warm and heavy.*
> *My legs are so relaxed that I can hardly feel them.*
> *My legs feel distant - almost as if they belong to someone else.*

My legs are distant and heavy.
Utterly relaxed.

By now, you should be starting to experience an overall feeling of calmness and relaxation. Continue to use this technique on the other major muscle groups in your body. Most people find this technique is most effective if they follow a rough anatomical pattern through their body, from legs to trunk, then to your arms, and finally to your head. For example, perform a two-breath cycle of relaxation on each of the following areas, just as you did for your leg muscles.

> *Tighten your tummy muscles ... relax.*
> *Arch your lower back slightly ... relax.*
> *Tighten your chest muscles ... relax.*
> *Pull your shoulder muscles up toward your ears ... relax.*
> *Tighten your upper arm muscles ...relax.*
> *Bend your hand back tightly at the wrist ... relax.*
> *Grip your fingers into a fist ... relax*

Once you have completed a contract-relax cycle for each of the above areas, reaffirm the relaxation of your whole trunk and arms, just

as you did with your whole leg area. Try
some phrases such as these.

> *Allow yourself to feel your torso and back.*
> *Feel the weight, heaviness and warmth of*
> *your back and torso.*
> *You feel so heavy that you are sinking into*
> *the floor or chair.*
> *Your body is so relaxed that you can no*
> *longer feel it.*
> *Feel the weight, heaviness and warmth of*
> *your arms.*
> *Your arms feel distant and unattached, like*
> *they belong to someone else.*
> *Your arms are relaxed, heavy and warm.*
> *They feel good to be so relaxed and calm.*

Finally, move to your neck, head and face
muscles.

> *Arch your neck slightly, then fully relax the*
> *back of your neck.*
> *Then tense the muscles at the front of your*
> neck (if you are lying, pretend to lift your
> head off the pillow) *then let it grow heavy.*
> *Concentrate on the heaviness of your head*
> *and neck.*
> *Slowly let your neck go loose, and feel the*
> *weight of your head.*

And then

> *Turn your attention to your cheeks.*
> *Feel the relaxation in your cheeks.*
> *Your cheeks are so utterly relaxed that you*
> *can feel the skin smoothing out.*
> *Your cheeks are heavy and smooth and*
> *relaxed.*

Repeat the above four line sequence for your jaw, then your forehead, your temples, and finally your eyelids.

At this stage you may wish to repeat a few deep relaxing breaths, and reaffirm your overall calmness and peacefulness. Next, move onto stage three, in which you will deepen your physical relaxation into mental relaxation.

(3) Mental relaxation

Now, you will use the relaxation of your facial area to induce a deep relaxation of your mind.

> *You can feel your eyelids resting gently on*
> *each other.*
> *Your eyelids feel heavy.*
> *Heavy and relaxed.*
> *Your whole face is relaxed.*

Relaxation right through your head.
Your whole head is relaxed.
Deeply relaxed.
Relaxed right through your mind.
Your mind is relaxed.
Your mind is heavy, warm and comfortable.

(4) Deepening your level of relaxation

You feel calm.
Calm and peaceful.
Utterly calm, all through your body.
Your whole body is relaxed.
Your mind and body are totally calm,
relaxed and peaceful.
You are so peaceful that your mind feels
light.
Your mind feels so light and relaxed that it
is starting to float.
You're mind is lightly floating.
Floating.
Your mind is drifting
Drifting.
Floating and drifting wherever it wishes to
go.
With each outward breath you grow even
more calm and peaceful.
Utterly peaceful.

At this point - if you're still reading - your mind should be fully calm and relaxed. Your thoughts will wander about of their own accord, like in a daydream. Do not attempt to control your thoughts, but instead just let them come and go as they wish. Don't try to pass judgements, or to solve any problems. Just relax, and enjoy the feeling of letting go.

If thoughts - especially worries or problems - enter your head, just *let them go*. It's as though your thoughts arrive on a bus, but do not get off. You simply let them pass through without evaluation, like passengers on a bus who do not alight.

Another useful analogy is to consider the thoughts as clouds drifting across the sky. Normally, you would focus on your thoughts, just as your eyes would normally focus upon the clouds. However, when you are deeply relaxed, you focus on the blueness of the sky, simply allowing the 'cloud-thoughts' to drift in and out of their own accord.

This final stage of deep mental relaxation is sometimes difficult for people to master. Sometimes, problems and worries just keep popping into your head. Fine. Let them. Let them drift in and out of your mind. *Just don't think about them.*

When you have mastered this art of letting go of thoughts, you will have truly arrived at a state of peace, calm and deep mental relaxation.

Now, you have one of three choices.

(1) Do nothing

You can simply stay in this state for a few minutes, gently experiencing the warm, comfortable feeling that comes with deep relaxation.

(2) Imagery or visualisation

You can use other techniques, such as imagery or visualisation, to help you achieve an even more deeply relaxed state.

For example, you may wish to imagine a passive scene from nature, such as a waterfall, a sunset, or gently rolling waves on a beach. Alternatively, you may wish to picture and experience yourself in a favourite imaginary place (it doesn't *have* to be a pub). Other people find that mental tricks, such as a cool wind blowing through their mind, can help to clear away feelings of tension or anxiety.

Some find that associating different colours - the colours of the rainbow, for example - with different calming emotions is useful. Then, when their mind is properly relaxed, they simply picture the colour, and automatically experience the relevant positive emotion. All of these 'tricks' are very simple yet effective.

Chapter five will outline some other ways in which you can use visualisation to help you achieve your goal of a pain-free life.

(3) You can use a technique known as *autosuggestion*.

As your brain is now wandering and relaxed, it is very receptive and uncritical of any ideas and thoughts that enter it. When in this accepting state, your brain will simply absorb any information that you supply it, without attempting to justify or analyse any instructions. You can then use this very useful state to help to alter your deepest perceptions and attitudes.

This area of mental exercise has many other names, including positive thinking,

affirmations and self-hypnosis, all of which
are essentially the same thing. These
strategies are so effective in achieving a wide
range of results, including decreasing your
pain, that we'll examine them in detail in the
next chapter.

(5) Return to wakefulness

After either performing visualisations,
autosuggestion or simply relaxing for a few
minutes, you are now ready to awaken back
to reality. There are no real secrets here. My
only suggestion is to arise slowly and
gradually, and keep the feelings of calmness
and peacefulness as you do.

Many people like to use an abbreviated,
reversed form of the progressive muscular
relaxation. This technique involves gently
feeling and moving your eyes, then your face
and neck. You then continue this pattern until
you have gently activated your arms, trunk,
legs and finally your feet.

Other people prefer a reverse counting
method. Here, you start counting at a number
such as twenty, subtracting one as you take
each inward breath. You gradually awaken

yourself as you count, so that as you hit zero you are fully awake, alert, refreshed and ready to go.

I hope that you now have a solid grounding in the skill of relaxation. Let's now look at another vital part of your mental approach to lower back pain: your attitude.

Chapter Five
"Attitudes, the placebo effect, and the power of the mind"

The health practitioner who resides within

Attitudes, the placebo effect and the power of the mind

Your attitude toward your pain has an enormous influence on your recovery. Many studies of recuperation rates from various maladies and illnesses show that your attitude is one of the most important factors in determining how much pain and suffering that you have to endure.

A widely accepted maxim in modern psychology is that 'where the mind goes, the body will follow'. If you understand and fully appreciate this idea, then you will have a huge advantage in your quest to get rid of your pain as quickly, easily and permanently as possible.

The principle of 'where the mind goes, the body will follow' can be seen at work in many spheres of human behaviour - especially in sport, where its effects are very apparent. For example, imagine two golfers - we'll call them Damian and Greg - on the last hole of a tournament, tied for the lead. As Damian tees up his ball, he realises that 250 metres away, on the left edge of the fairway, is a large, ominous sand bunker. In the back of his mind, Damian implores himself with the following instructions: 'Don't hit the ball into the bunker ... don't hit the ball to the left ... whatever you do, don't hook the ball....'

Soon, Greg is faced with the same shot. However, he gives his mind a different set of commands: 'Hit the ball onto the fairway ... hit the ball straight down the middle ... swing your club straight and true....'

Guess who won the tournament? Almost for sure, Greg would have walked away with the winner's cheque that day. Damian, having pictured the bunker in his mind so vividly, was very likely to have hit the ball straight into it. Greg peppered his mind with images of the middle of the fairway, which is probably where his ball landed.

Why do these results occur with such predicability? Simple: where the mind goes, the body will follow.

This effect was illustrated even more lucidly in one research study. The researchers connected an EMG machine - a device that measures the amount of electrical activity in a muscle - to the legs and arms of some elite downhill ski racers. The racers then imagined that they were skiing down a particular mountain, even though in reality they were lying perfectly still on the researchers table.

The EMG readings were then matched with the skiers' descriptions of their actions during the race. The results were uncannily accurate. Each time the skiers reported that they were visualising a jump, their leg muscles automatically increased their activity, ie. they performed a tiny contraction that was undetectable to the naked eye. The skiers arm muscles tightened ever so slightly as they imagined pushing with their stocks, while their leg muscles tightened appropriately during sharp turns.

The skiers' minds could not distinguish between a real experience and one that was vividly imagined. In short, the skiers muscles automatically followed and performed what their mind was visualising.

This reaction is not confined only to the sporting world. 'Where the mind goes, the body will follow' forms an inseparable part of our everyday life. For example, picture in your mind a person who is downhearted and depressed. Really try to visualise this person. Now, picture the same person in a joyful, happy mood. Consider this question: what posture did your imaginary person adopt in each situation?

Usually, a depressed mindset is associated with low muscle tone, a drooping head and a slumped back, while a happy, exuberant mind gives a decidedly more upright and buoyant posture. This difference illustrates that your muscles are influenced not only by your imagination, but by your mood as well!

Can you see that your state of mind has a huge effect on your physical body, not only during sporting events, but also in virtually every task that you attempt each day? In many different ways, your body reacts *automatically* to the images in your mind.

Guess what happens if you keep thinking about your pain? Think about that question, and apply the principle of 'where the mind goes, the body will follow'. The answer should be obvious: the more you think about your pain, the worse it will become.

Unfortunately, this mindset is exactly what most people tend to do. We tend to focus, dwell and worry about everything that is wrong, while ignoring the positive aspects of any situation.

Consider the following exercise. First, mentally list all the body parts with which you *don't* have any problems. For example, how are your elbows, your fingernails, the middle joint of your left little toe, your right kidney? What about diseases, such as polio, Paget's disease, paracoccidioidomycosis, or pachydermoperiostosis, just to name a few - count how many of those you *don't* have. Your lists, were they an exhaustive collection of all of your body parts and systems that work perfectly, would have millions of entries. Yet despite all of these wonderfully functioning, pain-free parts, you probably only concentrate on the parts that are sore, or don't work properly.

As you saw above, this preoccupation with your sore or stiff areas has one effect: it makes them worse. Are you starting to see why a positive attitude to your back pain is so important?

Pain can sometimes be difficult to ignore as it often causes reciprocal mental stress and tension. In more severe or prolonged cases, pain can also precipitate other mental states, such as agitation, anger, frustration and depression. These feelings increase your stress level, which then worsens the original problem. A vicious cycle can develop, which can be very difficult to break.

Often in these situations, the worry, resentment or brooding that comes with pain can cause more stress than does the physical injury. Not only that, but the *fear* of pain can be as debilitating, if not more so, than the pain itself. Some people live their lives never daring to do anything more challenging than watch television for fear of hurting themselves. This irrational fear is, in itself, a huge problem that seriously hinders recovery.

For all of the above reasons, a positive attitude to your pain is a vital part of your rehabilitation.

Does this all sound like bad news, and yet another problem that must be overcome if you are to relieve yourself of your pain? Despair not, for this effect works just as well in the forward, positive direction as it does in the backward, negative direction. In other words, if you can get your mind to believe that your troubles are resolving, then your body will follow it to health and well being. Your pain will magically disappear.

If this theory sounds a bit airy-fairy to you, or if it sounds like a wishy-washy dream of some alternate hippy therapists, then consider this fact: this power of the mind to cure the body is not only real, but is the most conclusively proven effect in the history of medical science.

I'll repeat that last sentiment again, in case you weren't paying attention. *The healing power of the mind over the body is the most conclusively proven effect in all of medicine.*

In medical and other health studies, it goes under the pseudonym of the *placebo effect*. Let's take a closer look at this interesting phenomenon, and see how you can use it to help cure your pain.

Whenever a new drug - or any other treatment, for that matter - is introduced, it must be tested on a large number of patients to see what effects, beneficial or harmful, it produces. Every good study then compares the results of the drug trial to what is known as a *placebo group*. This group, which is matched as closely as possible for conditions and symptoms to the medicated group, does not receive any real treatment. Instead, they receive a placebo treatment, which is a pill that has no effect whatsoever.

Usually, the placebo drug is a capsule that looks identical to the real drug, but is filled with nothing but harmless sugar. Of course, neither the control group nor the real group knows of the placebo. All subjects believe that they are taking a real drug.

Why do researchers go to this huge amount of trouble when they test a new drug or treatment? The reason is that those who take the placebo treatment always show a remarkable improvement as well!

Despite the fact that they have only swallowed a harmless sugar pill, many subjects in the placebo group report an improvement, sometimes even a complete cure, of their symptoms. In general, about 30% to 40% of people report an instant, seemingly miraculous cure following treatment that consists of absolutely nothing.

For example, in a study investigating the efficacy of new anti-inflammatory medication in eighty-eight arthritis sufferers, the same number of subjects reported relief following ingestion of a placebo as did patients who took the drug. Those patients who received no relief from the tablets were then given placebo injection. This theoretically useless injection cured 64% of the remaining difficult-to-cure cases!

Another study investigated the ability of a placebo drug to reduce post-surgical pain. One group of subjects were given intravenous doses of morphine - a very powerful pain-relieving drug - while the other group were given an intravenous placebo drug. The results showed that 52% of the patients on morphine experienced satisfactory pain relief, while the placebo group had satisfactory relief 40% of the time. In other words, the placebo was 77% as effective as morphine, one of the most powerful pain-relieving drugs available.

The placebo effect works in other ways. For example, a group of patients were given a placebo pill, but were told that it was a new antihistamine drug. Funnily enough, 77.4% of these patients reported a side effect of drowsiness, a common and well-known reaction to antihistamine medication.

For a placebo to work effectively, the patient must really believe that it will work. This effect was demonstrated in a study in which two groups of patients with ulcers were administered medication. The first group of subjects were told that the tablets contained a new drug that had been proven to drastically reduce the symptoms of stomach ulcers. Seventy percent of these patients reported significant relief from their symptoms. The members of the second group were told that their tablets contained a new experimental drug, whose effect on ulcers was largely unknown. Only 25% of these patients received adequate relief. But guess what? *Both* groups received identical tablets: a placebo!

I could continue to cite thousands of other studies that show the amazing ability of a placebo drug to cure an amazing array of illnesses. As mentioned earlier, the placebo affect is by far the most well proven theory in all of medical science.

How does a placebo create this wonderfully powerful healing effect? Possibly, some of the healing powers are due to *attribution:* the patient would have recovered anyway, but they attributed their improvement to the drug. However, this concept can not explain why many chronic patients, who have suffered with a serious ailment for years, suddenly recover when treated with placebo medication.

Many people have studied the placebo effect, trying to discover how it produces such amazingly powerful results. When all the hype, science and hoopla are stripped away, the answer is simple: it makes you *think positively*. The placebo drug creates an expectation in your mind that you will improve. Naturally, these positive thoughts and expectations soon become reality.

The placebo effect provides a wonderful illustration of the maxim with which we started this chapter: *where the mind goes, the body will follow.*

So how does this information apply to your pain? Well, if you can learn to create this placebo effect in yourself, you can reap the considerable, powerful benefits of this health practitioner who resides within your mind.

You have already seen how negative thinking and stress can produce damaging effects on your health and your pain level. You now know that positive thinking - which the placebo effect automatically creates - has overwhelmingly beneficial effects. Let's now learn how to turn damaging negative thoughts into positive expectations.

Getting rid of negative thinking

The first step to positive thinking is to rid yourself of negative, self-damaging thoughts and attitudes. This subject is obviously extremely complex; psychologists and psychiatrists spend years studying and treating this condition alone. However, you may find that the following information at least gets you thinking, as you may not even realise that you are carrying negative thoughts about your pain. For example, do any of the following situations ring true?

Have you ever....

- Moped about the house, feeling sorry for yourself, grumbling that your pain is ruining your day.

- Made your problems known to your friends, family and acquaintances, telling them all about your insufferable pain.

- Felt a sense of relief when your health practitioner diagnosed you with a 'serious problem'.

- Felt annoyed that no one else seems to care about your pain.

- Felt glad that your pain was allowing you time off from work, or other unpleasant tasks.

- Blamed someone else for causing your pain.

- Blamed a situation, such as a work task, or stressful situation, for your pain.

- Become frustrated that your injury has no blood, swelling or bruising with which you can prove to people that you are suffering.

- Tried some silly, medically unproven 'miracle' pill or treatment that was supposed to cure your condition.

Any of these thoughts familiar? If you sometimes think in any of these ways, then your mind, focusing on your problems, will soon start to drag your body down with it, causing even more pain, frustration and tension.

How do you avoid these negative thoughts? If you find yourself thinking this way, the first step is to ask yourself the following questions:

1. How do I feel at present?

We've already established that you feel frustrated, tense, fed-up and in pain.

2. How would I like to feel?

Naturally, most people would like to feel relaxed, calm, happy and pain free.

3. Are my thought patterns helping me to feel relaxed, calm, happy and pain free?

No, they are not. In fact, your negative attitude is clearly making your problem worse.

4. Then why am I doing something that makes me feel so bad?

This final question is by far the most important. Your honest answer will guide you to the best method for reversing your negative pattern of thought.

Note that you are not asking yourself why you have pain. This question has many answers, which a good health practitioner will help you to uncover. You are asking yourself why your *attitude* to your pain and disability is one that is clearly making you worse.

You don't have to pry deep into your childhood experiences and inner psyche to discover the answer. Just consider the question honestly.

By asking yourself these simple questions, you will see, in clear form, the basis of much of your negative thinking. Now let's see how to turn this negative, destructive attitude into a positive, helpful frame of mind.

Techniques for positive thinking.

Most of the following techniques can be used at any time. You can try them when you are in pain, in the car, on the toilet, or listening into the telephone while your Aunty Doris chatters unendingly about a dispute with her neighbours over the garbage bin. However, they are far more effective if you use them *regularly*, especially when performed *in conjunction with the relaxation exercises* that you learned in the last chapter.

As you know, a deeply relaxed mind does not criticise or analyse any new information that you present to it. Your mind simply accepts the thoughts as true, and automatically alters its attitudes and reactions. This effect is best seen during hypnosis, in which a hypnotist can convince a willing, hypnotised subject of the most absurd possibilities. Here, you will be using a similar technique known as *autosuggestion*.

For this reason, the instructions for these positive-thinking exercises are very simple. As with the relaxation exercises, your mind responds more readily to simple, straightforward statements than to complicated, detailed instructions. Please do not be discouraged by the seemingly simplistic nature of the following exercises. I urge you to try them, and you will soon see how effective they can be.

Affirmations

Affirmations are simply positive phrases that you repeat to yourself, either mentally or verbally. These phrases have an enormous effect on your mind, for while it is true that 'where the mind goes, your body will follow', it is equally true that 'where your speech goes, your mind will follow'. Therefore, you can control the reactions of your body just by thinking, or even saying, the right sentiments.

You can witness the power of affirmations in elite sporting situations. Phrases such as 'Come on, you can do it' are commonplace in virtually every sport, and represent the simplest, most basic form of an affirmation.

To apply this technique to your pain, you simply use positive phrases to convince your mind that you are well. Simply repeat the phrases for a few minutes, either silently to yourself, or audibly.

Remember, these phrases are far more powerful if you use them when your mind is in a deeply relaxed, receptive state.

Below are some examples of such phrases. You can pick a few of these that you feel will work for you, or you can create some of your own. However, ensure that the sentiments are positive, not a double-negative type phrase. Remember Damian the golfer, who told himself not to hit the ball in the bunker, but unerringly shot directly into the middle of the sand.

Examples of positive phrases

- I feel healthy and strong
- My body is calm and relaxed
- My back/head/leg feels wonderful
- I am strong, healthy and relaxed
- My muscles are loose and relaxed
- My whole body is 100% comfortable
- I feel confident and strong
- My back/leg/head will remain relaxed and healthy during any activity

Examples of phrases to avoid

- My back/leg/head does not hurt
- I cannot feel any pain
- I am not tense or tight
- I am not sick
- I do not feel any pain or tension

- My back/head/leg is pain free
- I will not retain any pain
- My pain will not hurt after lawn bowls today

Visualisation

As mentioned previously, your mind cannot distinguish between a real situation and one that you vividly imagine, as demonstrated by the champion skiers in the EMG study. You can use the technique of visualisation to help practice your attitudes and responses to many different situations.

I'm sure you've heard the old adage that 'practice makes perfect'. One Australian football coach refined this saying to *'perfect* practice makes perfect'. Luckily, you have a place in which you can practice perfectly every time: in your mind.

You can use the visualisation techniques to perfectly practice perfect responses to any situation that would previously have disturbed you.

The technique is, again, remarkably simple. During your *first* visualisation session, picture the problem in your mind. Then, after you have fully examined and experienced every detail of the picture, you abruptly change its polarity so that the situation is now as you would like it to be. In other words, you change the image so that it now depicts you solving your problem.

You then visualise this new, perfect picture for the ensuing few minutes, and in subsequent sessions. Never again should you visualise the picture containing the problem. Remember, your mind will go where your thoughts take it, so make sure that your thoughts are always showing the ideal situation, the solution.

Let's look at a few examples to see how visualisation can work.

Suppose that you feel extremely angry and tense each time your partner leaves their dirty clothes on the bathroom floor. Just the sight of the dirty jocks, socks and shirts makes your blood boil, and the subsequent stress gives you a burning headache for the next few hours. You've tried, you've really tried, to change your partner's habits, but no amount of berating, bribery or begging has made a difference. Instead, you decide to change yourself, by altering the way that you respond to the same situation.

To use a visualisation technique to help you overcome your stressful reaction, you would first picture yourself walking into the bathroom when your partner has left the floor covered with dirty clothes. See yourself becoming angry, and really experience the feelings of tension and frustration that your response brings. Vividly imagine the slowly ebbing head pain that grows with your tension levels.

Now, change the polarity of your vision. Again, picture yourself walking into the bathroom and seeing the filthy floor, but this time see yourself as being totally in control of your emotions. Really experience this new response. Feel the relaxation. Imagine yourself responding exactly as you would like. See yourself as calm, relaxed and with a clear head. Practice this response in your mind, and never again return to the old vision of a frustrated, angry, painful you.

After a few sessions, particularly if you combine this visualisation with your deep mental relaxation, you will find that this practiced response becomes your *natural reaction*. This may take up to six weeks, but if you practice this response diligently in your mind, then it will definitely happen. Never again will you feel stressed or pained by dirty clothes on the bathroom floor.

Note that you have not changed the external situation; you have simply changed how you respond to it.

You can also use this technique to practice physical responses. Many athletes visualise themselves successfully performing their chosen sport. Next time you are watching an elite sportsperson just before a competition, take note of their behaviour. Sometimes you can actually see them visualising every nuance of their performance.

One athlete who won an Olympic gold medal in middle distance running showed so little emotion after crossing the line in first place that friends later quizzed him on his lack of happiness. His reply was that he had already won the race thousands of times in his mind, and that this particular race was no different. He *knew* he was going to win. In fact, he was *bored* of winning that race. Visualisation can be very powerful.

Similarly, you can use visualisation to practice physical elements of your pain prevention program. For example, let's say that your back aches if you repeatedly lift with a poor technique. Unfortunately, your job as a supermarket grocery handler requires you to perform hundreds of lifts every day. In the rush and hustle of your work, your lifting technique often falters, and you find that your back pain is increasing as a result.

To help you with this aspect of your pain management, first perform your mental relaxation exercises. Then imagine yourself working frantically, behind schedule, with dozens of awkward lifts to complete before closing time. Visualise your lifting technique failing and your muscles flagging as you lose concentration. Feel your back pain increasing, and your stress level rising.

Now, change polarity. Imagine the same busy situation, but this time see yourself in control. Visualise your posture as perfect, and your lifting technique as infallible. Your muscles are firm, and your spine feels flexible and strong. Imagine that you easily complete all of your required lifts with ease, with no pain and no stress. Well done!

If you practiced and rehearsed this scene in your mind for a few weeks, the next time it arose you would respond exactly as you had 'practiced'. Remember, your mind cannot tell the difference between real and a vividly imagined situation. Perfect practice makes perfect.

Note that in both these situations, you practiced and visualised your response in advance. You cannot relax and visualise if you have already triggered frustrated emotions. For visualisation to be effective, you must train your mind *in advance* to replace the negative reactions with more favourable, automatic responses. In this way, you won't have to subdue any feelings of tension, because *they won't even occur*.

Five steps to prevent the onset of pain

The following technique was popularised by Bert Weir, an Australian stress control expert, as a treatment for migraine headaches. However, you can use it for almost any type of pain, particularly one that waxes and wanes over time. In fact, you could apply this exercise to any stress-related illness at all. The idea of the technique is to use relaxation, visualisation and affirmation techniques to banish any pain before it gets started.

Step One: As soon as you feel the first twinge of a pain, immediately stop what you are doing. Do not wait five minutes, for if you do a pain-tension-spasm-pain cycle may come into effect.

Step Two: Perform your relaxation exercises. In the beginning, this may take you up to half an hour. However, with practice you should be able to achieve a suitably relaxed mind within five minutes.

Step Three: Slowly work through the following positive phrases

> *I can feel pain coming on*
> *I do not want pain*
> *I do not deserve pain*
> *I want my (head/back/leg) to remain relaxed, comfortable and healthy*

My (head/back/leg) is relaxed, comfortable and healthy

<u>Step Four:</u> Come out of your relaxation phase, and undertake a different activity than what you were doing when the pain started. At the very least, you should assume a different posture.

<u>Step Five:</u> If the twinge of pain returns, then immediately repeat the whole process.

A brief reminder ...

In this chapter, you have seen how your mind has remarkable subconscious control over your body. The well-proven placebo effect illustrates the powerful positive effect that your mind possesses over even extreme pain. You have learned some simple techniques to turn your negative thought processes into positive feelings, and so generate healing and health.

Chapter Six

"Over to you!"

Over to you!

I'm sure that you'll benefit from the techniques that you have learned in this booklet. Relaxation, visualisation and positive thinking are the most natural of all cures, yet, as thousands of studies have shown, are among the most powerful.

Hopefully, you can now see that

- Stress is rife in modern society, and many people are overly stressed without even realising it.

- The fight-or-flight response, which is the body's natural reaction to stress, is an inappropriate yet unavoidable response to stressful situations

- If your body is frequently or constantly in a low-grade fight-or-flight response, it can suffer from a widespread array of health problems

- The fight-or-flight response can cause joint or muscular pain, arthritis, and can also heighten your perception of pain

- To decrease the effects of stress you can either…

(a) Increase your tolerance to stress, by living a healthy lifestyle

(b) Remove or change the things that are stressing you, which may or may not be practical

(c) Change yourself, by practicing deep mental relaxation exercises, so that you are no longer bothered by things that would once have stressed you

- Your mental attitude to your problem has a great influence on your recovery rate. Remember, where the mind goes, the body will follow, so if you continue to focus on your pain, it will worsen.

- If you believe that your pain will go away, it probably will. This is known as the placebo effect, and is the most conclusively proven theory in all of medical science

- By allowing your mind to enter a deeply relaxed state, it becomes receptive and uncritical. When you are deeply relaxed, you can easily convince yourself that your pain is disappearing.

- By visualising and practicing your response to known stressful situations, you can avoid feelings of tension and pain even starting.

You've learned a lot about stress, relaxation, positive thinking and visualisation, haven't you? With some dedicated practice, I'm sure that you will quickly master the techniques and suggestions. Of course, you shouldn't expect the changes to occur overnight. But with some gentle daily persistence, even the most chronically overstressed and uptight person can achieve unbelievable results within a month or two.

You will soon find that your days will more relaxed and pain free than ever before. Your productivity and health will improve, and you'll notice many beneficial side effects. And because you've taken the time to learn the skills of relaxation, the techniques will stay with you for life. In short, you have learned how to use your brain to get rid of your pain.

Good luck!

More books by John Perrier
from JP Publishing Australia

"Back Pain: How to get rid of it Forever"

- Self help/back pain/self treatment
- Adult/Young Adult readers
- Available as print edition or two-volume E-Book

"Captain Rum – A Wondrous Adventure"
Edited by Prof. H.D. (Bert) Lampluck

- Historical Fiction/Maritime adventure
- Adult/Young Adult readers
- Published by JP Publishing Australia
- Available as print or E-Book

"A Few Quiet Beers with God"

- Science-fiction/comedy
- Young Adult/Teen/Young-at-heart adults
- Available as print or E-Book

"Campervan Kama Sutra"

- Travel/comedy
- Young adult/Adult
- Available as print or E-book

You can find more online at
www.JPpublishingAUSTRALIA.com

"Back Pain: How to Get Rid of it Forever"

The title says it all: this book will help you permanently banish your back pain. In three logical sections (or two E-book volumes) it shows you how to feel better.

The first section makes it easy for you to understand your back pain. Using simple, clear language, it explains the structure of your spine, and demystifies many common pain-provoking conditions. The second part offers a unique quiz that will help you to classify your injury into one of four types. In this way, you will learn how to cure your pain, not someone else's.

In part three, the advice flows thick and fast. You will learn clever techniques that will help you to use your spine more efficiently, and discover how to think, eat, relax, and sleep away your pain. You'll also find useful information on exercises, x-rays, medication and muscles, plus some tips on how to choose a spinal health practitioner. Of course, all of the advice will be tailored to your specific problem.

Because the cure uses well-proven techniques, your relief won't just last a few days or weeks. You will feel better *forever*.

More information on *Back Pain* can also be found at www.physioworks.com.au

"Captain Rum: A Wondrous Adventure"
Edited by Prof. H.D. (Bert) Lampluck

When an Oxford Professor stumbles upon an old naval Captain's log, he unwittingly discovers what many scholars now agree is one of the greatest maritime adventures in history.

In 1821, Captain Fintan McAdam set sail from London, solo, in search of adventure. During his journey he discovered incredible new worlds, and interacted with their amazing inhabitants. McAdam's voyage also forced him to confront his enemies within, learning much about himself.

Captain Rum, as told in McAdam's own words through his journal, is a tale of discovery, despair and delight. It will keep you enthralled through many a stormy night.

"A Few Quiet Beers with God"

Set in Australia in the year 2031, this story is science-fiction comedy at its best.

When Dave, a hopeless but lovable 34 year old, meets Alexandra, the girl of his dreams, he feels as though his luck has finally changed. But due to his ineptness with technology, he tragically loses contact with her.

Meanwhile, the lust for supremacy of two powerful Americans ignites a bitter feud. Their fight reaches around the globe and soon entwines not only Dave and Alexandra, but also a superstar football player nicknamed 'God'.

Their final meeting precipitates an event that no-one saw coming.

"Campervan Kama Sutra"
Outback Australia, with a camper trailer, three kids and a dog*.

This true story tells of one family's hilarious journey through Australia's rugged outback countryside.

Our intrepid adventurers work their way through numerous mishaps, including, but not limited to, an ill-advised river crossing, an inappropriately packed roof rack and some truly horrible singing.

During their journey they stumble across a motley assortment of characters such as a confused check-in clerk, a grey nomad with an eye for detail regarding torches, and several Crazy Germans.

While reading *Campervan Kama Sutra*, you'll not only fall in love with Australia's vast, ever-changing countryside, but you'll also delight in the tragicomedy that arrives with unerring regularity. You'll laugh until something hurts.

*P.S. There was no dog.

Connect and Contact

Your comments, criticisms, typos, praise and suggestions are all very welcome. Please contact us by any of the methods below.

Email
JDPpublishingAUSTRALIA@gmail.com
(please note the extra 'D')

Facebook
https://www.facebook.com/JPpublishingAustralia

Website
www.JPpublishingAUSTRALIA.com

Mail
JP Publishing Australia
56 Quirinal Crescent
Seven Hills, Brisbane
AUSTRALIA   4170

www.ingramcontent.com/pod-product-compliance
Lightning Source LLC
Chambersburg PA
CBHW060907280326
41934CB00007B/1222